# IIFYM: If It Fits Your Macros

## The Ridiculously Simple Guide to Losing Weight Without Giving Up Your Favorite Foods

### Christian Pinedo

**Disclaimer**

This book is for informational purposes only. Use of the guidelines in this book is a choice of the reader. This book is not intended for the treatment or prevention of disease. This book is also, not a substitute for medical treatment or an alternative to medical advice.

# Contents

# The FREE IIFYM Bonus Companion Course

To help guide you through this book, I created a free bonus companion course. The course includes more tutorials, downloadable worksheets and materials, a ton of bonus materials, and all the resources and links mentioned in the book. Your first step in succeeding with IIFYM is signing up for this free course. The course makes it easy for you to find what you need as you read along. Visit the following link to get the free bonus companion course now:

## *iifymbook.club*

Also, if you have any questions or run into any problems, shoot me an email at chris@leanwithstyle.com and I'll do my best to help!

**Thanks,**
**Christian Pinedo**

# Introduction
# Who is Christian Pinedo?

I'm Christian, and my mission is to show people how to achieve the body of their dreams without sacrificing their favorite foods.

For over a decade now, I've been experimenting and learning about what works and what doesn't when it comes to getting lean.

And, I can confidently say, while I'm not the strongest or leanest individual on the planet, I know what works and what doesn't.

But it wasn't always this way. You see, I was a fat, out of shape, kid growing up. How fat was I, you might be wondering?

Well, keep reading to see just how fat I really was (don't worry, there'll be pictures soon):

My mother, bless her heart, was on her way home when I had called and asked if I could have two Big Mac sandwiches (yes, two) with a large fry and large coke (I know, I know).

She had denied my wishes and, obviously, I started fighting and crying over the phone. Eventually, she gave in and I was at home waiting for her arrival. My mom, who was only looking out for my health, only ordered one Big Mac.

Two was outrageous for a teenager/kid (really no kid that age should be eating Big Macs, but that's a different debate for another time).

When I noticed that she had only ordered one Big Mac, I threw the biggest fat-boy tantrum you can only imagine.

I must have whined and cried for 10 minutes, after finishing the single Big Mac of course. I was *so upset that my mother didn't give me two Big Macs.*

*My mother gave me the biggest whopping ever that day and rightfully so.*

*(So, that's how fat I was.)*

I like to joke around with my friends that my fat-boy tantrum was just like the scene in Breaking Bad (best show ever) from the episode *Crawl Space*. If you've watched Breaking Bad, you know exactly what freak-out scene I'm talking about.

Anyways, that was me. Fat and out of shape growing up.

Not only that but my nickname throughout my childhood was "Potato."

Seriously.

*They called me Potato (still am by my close friends) all throughout middle school and high school.*

Back in 6th Grade, my teacher couldn't pronounce my last name "Pinedo".

I told him how to say it (pin-a-doe), and he said:

**"Oh. That sounds like Potato."**

And thus, my nickname, Potato, was born.

*I'm also brown and I was chubby back then...so, that didn't help.*

Later on, throughout high school, when people called me Potato, it wasn't in a "bullying" fashion.

People REALLY called me that (I'm sure some who didn't know me were trying to put me down, but I didn't pay attention).

**I can't tell you how many people during those years came up to me and asked me what my real name was.**

They only knew me as Potato.

When I told them, my name was actually Christian, they said *"Yeah, no that doesn't sound right."* *Throws hands in air*

So, I stopped trying to correct people and so I just went with it.

Anyways, it wasn't until High School that I started a semi-structured workout routine. That's because I was playing high-school football and my quest to getting fit and losing weight had begun.

Like most newbies, I had no idea what I was doing. I just followed coaches' orders, and so did everyone else. I had no idea about nutrition or if the workouts we were doing were optimal for strength and aesthetics.

During the football season, I was in kind of good shape (I played left guard on the offensive line for anyone who cares). However, when that offseason hit, it was back to fat Christian.

It got worse when football (and High School) had ended. I ballooned up to 235 lbs. during the end of my senior year. During football, I was 180 lbs. at my lowest but averaged 200 lbs. throughout high school.

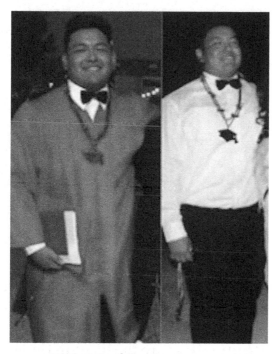

*High School Graduation 2013*

After I saw my graduation pictures, I was disgusted. I promised myself to get "serious" about this whole weight loss thing and to get lean.

And, here's the 2.5 year "transformation" picture:

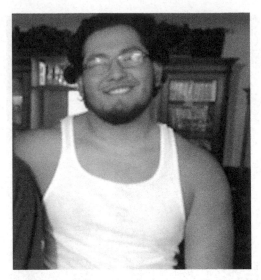

*January 2015 (Look at that hair! Who let me out of the house!)*

**Just pathetic.** Here are the types of things I had read and believed during those 2.5 years:

- "Avoid carbs if you want to lose weight!"
- "Don't eat rice. Rice makes you fat!"
- "Don't eat before bed."
- "I heard fruit is bad for you, so I don't eat fruit anymore."
- "Keto is the only way to lose weight."

- "Calories don't matter. Just eat 5-7 meals a day with 2 hours of each other to boost your metabolism."

I know I shouldn't have, but I took these recommendations as fact. I still hear this sh** thrown around today. It's just silly.

I spent two years following sh** advice from magazine articles, bodybuilding dot com workouts, and straight-up fitness scammers.

I tried many different dieting and training techniques. I tried personal training at my local gym, and they just had more of the same sh** advice as the magazine articles and forums did.

I've spent hundreds (probably thousands) of dollars on online fitness courses and programs.

After all that time, I knew what brought the most results, and what brought close to nothing.

I want to save you as much time as possible, so you don't have to take more than 2 years to see fat loss success as I did and that's what this book is all about.

After almost a year of following and learning about IIFYM and nutrition, I lost about 50 pounds:

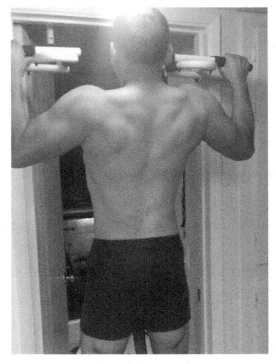

*December 2015*

Needless to say, I was thrilled.

I accomplished my goal, and set new ones, after this picture. That was to help as many people get through all the noise and B.S. out there in the fitness space.

This is my most recent "physique update" picture:

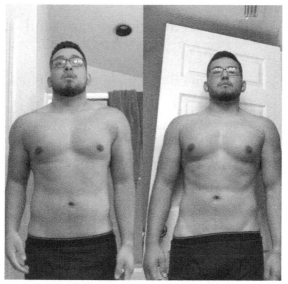

*2019, End of bulk (left) – End of Cut (right)*

I don't have the greatest physique and I'm not the strongest, nor do I claim to be.

What I do claim to know is how to show you how to get lean without giving up your favorite foods or going on any strange diet. All it takes is some planning, hard work, and dedication. Let's go to it.

# The Key Messages of This Book

If at any point in this book you feel overwhelmed, refer to this section because it outlines the truth and that is this:

- You don't need to give up carbs and sugar to lose weight
- You don't need to eat clean (e.g., chicken, broccoli, and brown rice) every day to get or stay lean
- You don't need any fat burners, fat blockers or any other supplements for weight loss
- You don't need to eat something every couple of hours to boost your metabolism
- You don't need to starve yourself to lose weight

As you'll see in this book, *IIFYM: If It Fits Your Macros*, I'll keep things simple. Too many fitness books try to cover every little thing about fat loss leaving you with an unread book because it's just all too much.

I want you to finish this book as fast as possible, and then, **take action**. Therefore, you will see action steps to take at the end of each chapter or section, and they will help get you started. These steps, along with the free companion course, will make you successful.

**With that said, here are the key messages of my book:**

- Your caloric intake is what determines whether you lose weight or gain weight. That's it. If you want to lose weight, lower your calories. Vice versa if you want to gain weight.
- Your macronutrient intake (or "split") is what determines where the majority of that weight you lose (or gain) comes from or as.
- Because macronutrients (macros for short) have their caloric makeup, tracking your macros is the same as tracking calories (I will show proof later in the book). Thus, by tracking macros, you are also tracking

calories which, as we know, determines your weight loss or gain.

- Instead of *only* having a calorie limit each day, you will also have a macronutrient limit each day.

- You can have whatever foods you'd like so long as you don't go over this macro limit each day. This strategy is called IIFYM: If It Fits Your Macros (is it starting to make sense?).

- So yes, you can lose weight, get lean, build muscle, while eating foods you actually like and without giving up carbs or fats or anything!

This all may sound like hoopla at the moment, but throughout the book, you will learn exactly how and why following IIFYM is the best way to lose fat and get lean in an enjoyable way.

You'll also notice that there is no simple secret or hack that I am going to describe to you in this book. **That's because there isn't one.** I used to think there was one, but there isn't. It just takes hard work and dedication.

I'm going to show you exactly how to do everything I just mentioned above and more. Again, the companion course is there to walk you through the process step-by-step. You can get access to it for free with the following link:

**iifymbook.club**

If I could hope for one thing from this book, it would be that you become a master of IIFYM and learn the basics of nutrition. The goal of this book is not to teach you about everything under the sun about nutrition. Only the key points that you need to know to get lean.

I hope that you then apply these skills to your own life and start teaching others around you. Perhaps it will be helping your workout partner or significant other lose weight by showing them what you learned in this book.

Whatever it is, I hope this book helps you reach your ultimate goal in your fitness journey, and I wish you the best.

**To Your Success,**
**Christian Pinedo**

# Chapter 1
# What Is IIFYM?

*"Take care of your body. It's the only place you have to live."*

*- Jim Rohn*

IIFYM is a method, or style, of dieting used to improve body composition by tracking your macronutrients (macros). IIFYM stands for "If It Fits Your Macros." There are three main macros that are traditionally accounted for: protein, carbs, and fats. By tracking these macros on your fitness goal pursuit, you'll naturally be tracking your calories as well. Why does that matter?

If you've done any research on IIFYM in the past, perhaps you've realized that no foods are off limits and that no food groups are labeled as good or bad for you. What matters in this style of dieting is **IF** your daily macro budget has room for the foods you want to eat. If so then you're in the clear; more on this soon.

Contrary to popular belief, IIFYM is NOT about eating Pop-Tarts for breakfast every day. Unlike traditional diets, you have the *option* to eat what you want, when you want, if you make it fit into your daily macro budget.

Although the option to eat junk food (pizza, burgers, ice cream, cookies, etc.) exists, you certainly **don't** have to partake in it. The *edge* that IIFYM dieting has over traditional dieting is its flexibility. This flexibility offers you the ability to improve your body composition without having to be perfect with your diet.

The bottom line on IIFYM: it offers anyone the opportunity to **tailor** their diet to include their favorite nutritious foods while mixing their favorite treats every day — and still making progress towards their fitness goals.

## Why Being Strict With Your Diet Is Not The Answer

Is it realistic to say that you're never going to eat ice cream, burgers, or pizza again? Are your only carbs going to come from veggies? (I can't even stand the thought.) Are you really going to trade all these so-called "dirty foods" out for meals consisting of chicken, brown rice, broccoli, and maybe some sweet potatoes if you're lucky?

My guess is probably not. That approach to weight loss causes all-out binge days or late-night cravings. Not only would your diet be strict and boring, but you'll most likely gain back all the "strict diet" weight you lost in the first place because it was unsustainable from the start. IIFYM on the other hand **IS** sustainable. This is very common with fad diets that severely limit a specific macronutrient (usually fat or carbs).

A study done found that when it comes to diets, people who try sticking to super strict diets were more prone to eating disorders, they carried more body fat, and they were also generally more depressed and miserable.[1]

The best fat loss approach — in my experience and for thousands of others — has been IIFYM. Another name for this revolutionary way of eating is *Flexible Dieting*. In this book, I'll be using these two names interchangeably. And although IIFYM can be used to gain lean muscle mass, in this book, we're focusing on IIFYM for fat loss (I'll still go over examples for bulking). This approach to fat loss will allow for realistic and long-lasting results.

## Beyond Weight Loss Benefits

Is IIFYM superior to most diets? A legion of flexible dieters will answer "yes," but the benefits of flexible eating exceed the weight loss realm. Here are more benefits of the IIFYM lifestyle.

## Realistic & Psychologically Beneficial

With flexible dieting, you don't have to make crazy lifestyle adjustments that involve buying ingredients you've never heard of before. You get to stick with the foods you love and lose weight while doing so!

Moreover, people enjoy the flexibility IIFYM offers while on their weight loss journeys, an unheard-of concept before discovering flexible dieting. This is especially true among women. In a study by Pennington Biomedical Research Center, 188 women were studied to see how they react to flexible dieting versus a traditional rigid diet. Here's what they found:

*"The study found that individuals who engage in rigid dieting strategies reported symptoms of an eating disorder, mood disturbances, and excessive concern with body size/shape. In contrast, flexible dieting strategies were not highly associated with BMI, eating disorder symptoms, mood disturbances, or concerns with body size."*

Mood disturbances? Any of those other symptoms ring any bells? No wonder there were so few people who actually got results with rigid fad diets.[2]

## A Long-Term Approach To A Healthy Lifestyle

Flexible dieting is about balance. You won't be giving up potatoes because carbs are the "enemy" and they are not the reason you can't lose weight. IIFYM encourages a balanced macronutrient intake giving your body the nutrients it requires to function efficiently. This is a much better and healthier approach to weight loss and has long term health benefits.

## It's Derived From Science-Based Weight Loss Principles

We'll discuss this in more detail in chapter two, but basically, flexible dieting follows universal laws. These laws have been proven time and time again and cannot be ignored in terms of fat loss. There is no manipulating these laws to your benefit. The best you can do is follow them to achieve your desired outcome. And that's exactly what IIFYM accomplishes if followed correctly.

## You Can Track Your Way To Success

Tracking your macros has never been easier. *My Fitness Pal* (MFP) has the capability of tracking your meals and equating them to calories and macros. You can easily adjust meals with this app and adjust what you've consumed in real-time. Furthermore, apps like MFP keep daily logs of prior day entries so you can easily add what you ate yesterday without having to re-enter meals each day. It's a powerful, free tool that is perfect for flexible dieters. More on tracking and MFP soon.

## Two Common Misconceptions Of IIFYM

Before you start IIFYM, get clear on the most common IIFYM misconceptions so you can experience the most success from it.

**Misconception #1: IIFYM Is Just an Excuse to Eat Junk Food Every Day**

This is inarguably the most common misconception associated with flexible dieting. This fad started on social media when the hype surrounding IIFYM was at its peak. Posts of cake, pizza, doughnuts and other types of junk on Facebook and Instagram under the hashtag #IIFYM and #flexibledieting created this notion. However, IIFYM is not just about eating junk, but it is how the lifestyle is marketed sometimes.

IIFYM is simply about giving people flexibility when it comes to their food choices. This flexibility *does* include treating yourself and it can be done daily if setup correctly. Where things go wrong (usually with beginners) is when people take IIFYM to the extreme, eating junk food because it "fits their macros." In actuality, eating an all-out junk diet is extremely unhealthy and impedes your weight loss or bodybuilding goals. Have you tried eating nothing but junk food all day? Chances are you never truly feel full and satiated, and you are always thinking of your next fast food meal.

The majority of people who practice IIFYM are **educated dieters** who understand nutrition. Truly understanding and practicing IIFYM entails understanding the basics of macronutrients. My goal with this book is to have you join the ranks of the educated IIFYM community.

## Misconception #2: IIFYM Is A Diet

Some think IIFYM is another diet with radical ideas. However flexible dieting is not really a diet but simply a nutritional and science-based approach to changing body composition. The human body needs specific amounts of nutrients to function efficiently every day. IIFYM lets you choose nutritious foods you like and there's room for treating yourself, all provided you stick to your macro targets. Don't expect strict diet recipes or limitations on your foods here.

Now that you have a better idea of what IIFYM is and know the misconceptions of IIFYM, we're ready to cover the fundamentals that you'll need to know to implement IIFYM into your daily routine. Spoiler alert: it all starts with calories.

# Chapter 2
# The Fundamentals of Calories

*"Everything is energy, and that's all there is to it. Match the frequency of the reality you want, and you cannot help but get that reality. It can be no other way. This is not philosophy. This is physics."*
*- Albert Einstein*

Weight loss is simple. The explanation of weight loss boils down to universal laws: The Laws of Thermodynamics in our case. These laws are traditionally open and closed systems, however, they can be used to explain biological open systems like you and me.

The First Law of Thermodynamics simply states that energy can neither be created nor destroyed and is often referred to as The Law of Energy Balance (or energy balance law). The human body similarly obeys this law.

$$(\text{Change in Internal Energy}) = (\text{Heat}) - (\text{Work})$$

This law gets the credit for how much weight we lose or gain. There is no debate on this. This is fact. A calorie, by definition, is a unit of heat energy.

If we eat more than our body requires every day, we can expect to gain weight. Gaining weight typically means the body is in a **caloric surplus**. The result is usually unwanted fat stores from too much energy entering our system.

On the other hand, if you eat less than your body needs every day, you can expect to lose weight. Losing weight is attributed to being in a **caloric deficit**.

Our bodies can also be at equilibrium, meaning our weight remains the same. In this case, the body is at a **caloric maintenance** level.

When the energy balance equation is applied to health and fitness, it simply translates to energy (foods) that enters the body and energy that leaves the body as either work (exercise) or heat. This is what the formula looks like when applied to weight change:

$$(\text{Change in Body Weight}) = (\text{Energy Consumed}) - (\text{Energy Expended})$$

If I know one thing for certain, it's this: **numbers don't lie**. And if you're anything like me, you want to know that you're on the right track with your weight loss goals. I don't like guessing by eyeballing portions and HOPING I'm in a caloric deficit. There's no need to drag out the weight loss process. Tracking your macros will take you a long way as they track your calories by default. (You'll see why in the next chapter.)

Food tracking apps like MFP make tracking calories and macro consumption a breeze.

Here's what I mean:

| 2,000 | - | 0 | + | 0 | = | 2,000 |
| Goal | | Food | | Exercise | | Remaining |

Look familiar? That's because it's the energy balance equation in action, slightly rearranged in MFP.

## Calories and Weight Loss

Scientific estimates place a pound of fat around 3,500 calories. If you want to lose a pound of fat, you have to eat 3,500 calories **less** every week. The 3,500 calories, over the span of a week, comes from your daily caloric deficit (500 calories x 7 days).

This is why exercise is a supplemental activity to being in a caloric deficit; it helps weight loss because you're expending more energy — along with eating less than normal. When it comes to the weight loss, success is 80% food intake and 20% physical activity. These numbers are not exact, **but can you see how it's easier to NOT eat a banana that's 100 calories than it is to burn 100 calories on a cardio machine?**

On average, a male requires 2,500 calories per day to maintain a healthy weight and around 2,000 calories to lose around a pound of fat weekly. On average a female requires 2,000 calories daily to maintain a stable weight and 1,500 calories to lose up to a pound a week.

You might've heard of these estimates before, right? These are just estimates, yet some people follow them and don't see results because they don't account for their size, health condition, current weight, age, gender, levels of physical activity, and so on.

**Calculating Your Caloric Deficit**

Now that you know that the key to tipping the weight scale in your favor involves being in a caloric deficit, here's how you calculate your caloric deficit (i.e., the number of calories you have to eat to lose one to two pounds per week).

To determine your caloric deficit, we must first calculate maintenance calories, also known as Total Daily Energy Expenditure (TDEE).

You can calculate your maintenance calories by using the following formula. (Note: this is just one of many ways to calculate your maintenance calories.)

| Maintenance Calories (or TDEE) = | (*14 or 16*) x body weight (lbs.) |
|---|---|

**Note:** *the formula above is just one of many ways to get your TDEE/maintenance calories. It assumes 1 hour of exercise plus normal daily activity and takes into account the following four factors: resting metabolic rate, thermic effect of activity, thermic* *effect of food, and non-exercise activity thermogenesis.[3]*

*It's important to note that any online calculator or different formula are at best estimations. The purpose of them are to give us starting points for individuals to test out. Feel free to use another tool to determine your TDEE if you're not comfortable using this multiplier method.*
*In chapter 4, we'll do more examples that involve distributing macros among your caloric deficit.*

The multiplier varies for men and women. For women, it's 14 calories/lb. since their metabolism is normally slower. For men, it's 16 calories/lb. There are a lot more to these multipliers than just adjusting for metabolism. One of the first flexible dieting authorities, Lyle McDonald, introduced this approximation formula. The keyword being "approximation." Which is what you need to get the ball rolling in the right direction.

Here's what Lyle said about his formula:

*"In general, women or those with a 'slower' metabolic rate should use the lower value (14 cal/lb.) and men or those with a 'faster' metabolic rate should use the higher value (16 cal/lb.) as a STARTING POINT ESTIMATION for maintenance calories.*

*By the way, slower and faster above are sort of subjective decisions, usually based on previous dieting and relatively tendency to gain or lose weight. It simply represents inherent variability in the components of total energy expenditure."*

Because these are Starting Point Estimations, **I've changed the formula to range from 14 TO 16 instead of 14 OR 16**. Go ahead and calculate your Maintenance Calories now:

| 14 - 16 x B.W. = | _____ x _____ lb. = | _____ Maintenance Calories (TDEE) |
|---|---|---|

Now that we have our Maintenance Calories, what

you want to next is subtract twenty to twenty five percent from your maintenance calories and you'll get your caloric deficit numbers.

| Calorie Deficit = | Maintenance Calories – (20 OR 25%) |
|---|---|

Another simple way to calculate caloric deficit is using this equation.

| Calorie Deficit = | Maintenance Calories x (.80 OR .75) |
|---|---|

Choosing between 25% or 20% is up to you. If you're looking for a more aggressive weight loss approach, choose 25%.

**Let's take a female that weighs 160 lbs**. At this weight, her approximate maintenance calories are 2,240 calories using the 14 calories/lb. multiplier (from earlier).

| 14 x 160 lbs. = | 2240 Maintenance Calories |
|---|---|
|  |  |

And her daily caloric deficit is 1,792 calories. Here's how we got that:

| Calorie Deficit for 160 lb. Female = | 2240 x .80 = | 1792 Calories |
|---|---|---|

Assuming this individual loses one to two pounds per week for the first two months and wants to lose an additional five to ten pounds she may need to adjust her caloric deficit again.

She would do this by repeating this calculation above (starting from maintenance calories) with her new weight. In other words, eventually everyone hits stagnation. *We'll cover what to do in that situation later.*

First, we need to bring in macros into the mix. Remember, the Law of Energy Balance (The First Law of Thermodynamics) when applied to biological systems is only about weight; it doesn't take into account *where* that weight comes from. This is where the effect of macronutrients on body composition comes into play.

# Exercise – Free Bonus Companion Course

To make this chapter really stick, I made a quick lesson showing you other ways on how to calculate your calorie deficit based on your activity levels. In the lesson we go over the following:

- Bob – 'Very Active' Example

- Pablo – 'Sedentary' Example

- Bob vs Pablo - Why being sedentary is Dangerous

- Ashley – 'Lightly Active' Example


I go over all of these examples in your course. These are all in Part 1 of your bonus IIFYM Companion course, which you can gain access to at:

## *iifymbook.club*

# Chapter 3
# Macronutrients and Body Composition

*"You should measure things you care about. If you're not measuring, you don't care, and you don't know."*

*– Steve Howard*

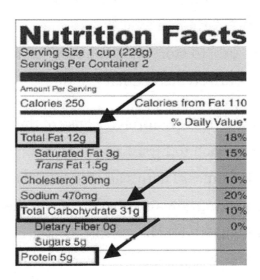

Macronutrients are essential when it comes to body composition, diet satiety, and adherence. Macronutrients, scientifically, involve the Second Law of Thermodynamics and deals with entropy.

The Second Law states that it's impossible for a system to consume energy and have an equivalent amount of work as a result. **In other words, in terms of body composition, a calorie is not a calorie.** We know this is true because it's proven that each macronutrient has different thermic effects on the body. When you eat food, your digestive system requires different levels of energy, depending on the macronutrients in your meal, to break them down. It costs energy to digest, absorb, to store those nutrients. Thus, not all calories are created equal.

Macros are usually ignored because of the "tunnel vision" approach to First Law of Thermodynamics. There's an overemphasis on calorie consumption and not enough on macro consumption, which plays a role in your body's composition. Neglecting a macronutrient — take protein for instance — can lead to losing weight from lean muscle mass instead of body fat stores. Such phenomena can occur when you only focus on calories in versus calories out and forget about the three essential macronutrients and their nutritional roles. **If macronutrients are neglected for too long, metabolism deteriorates over time, which is not an ideal case for anyone.**

Keeping track of macronutrient consumption, specifically the percentage of each, makes your fat loss journey healthy and enjoyable. Because you're giving your body the right number of macros your body needs, you'll feel full and satiated even in a caloric deficit. **Despite what you might have heard, being in a caloric deficit doesn't have to be a miserable experience or an overwhelming test of your willpower!**

Before we get to macronutrient calculations, let's make sense of how macros will play a role in your caloric deficit.

# Macros 101

## Protein

### *(1 gram of protein = 4 calories)*

The building blocks of proteins are amino acids, which are responsible for repairing and building muscle tissue. There are two types:

- Essential amino acids

- Nonessential amino acids.

The body can manufacture the nonessential amino acids, and it relies on you to feed it the essential amino acids (which come in the form of protein).

Protein tends to be the most commonly neglected macronutrient and usually takes a backseat behind carbs and fats. This is backwards thinking! There are good reasons not to neglect protein.

First, protein-rich foods provide satiety, which decreases the feeling of hunger when you're a few hundred calories below maintenance.[4] In fact, a study from the Department of Foods and Nutrition at Purdue University studied both young and old men to examine how their appetite responds to habitual protein intakes. The study found that both younger and older men who **consumed insufficient amounts of protein** experience appetite changes that can involve an excess in food intake.

Second, multiple studies show that protein has the greatest thermic effect out of the three macros.[5] Meaning, eating protein takes more energy (calories) to digest, absorb, and store than carbs or fats. You're burning more calories when you eat protein.

Here's a list of some major quality protein sources:

- Meat and poultry
- Fish (salmon, tuna, tilapia, etc.)

- Dairy Products (milk, yogurt, cottage cheese, etc.)

- Whole eggs and egg whites

- Lentils

- Legumes

- Quinoa

These quality proteins will ensure you're getting your essential amino acids replenished. Add them to your meal schedule — we'll get into examples of those soon — and you won't have a problem hitting your daily protein macro target.

Note: For Vegan protein sources and other recommendations, I highly recommend reading this informative article on the topic from Mike Matthews. You can find it at the following link:

### *bit.ly/vegan-ps*

# Carbohydrates

## (1 gram = 4 calories)

Carbs provide the body with the fuel needed for everyday living and help you feel energized throughout the day. They are the essential, must have, fuel source for every cell in the body. Carbs also aid in the digestion and utilization of proteins and fat. The body prefers carbs for energy because it's the one macronutrient that is most efficiently turned into energy.

This macro is especially vital for fitness enthusiasts and maximal sports performance. And even if you're not a professional athlete and regularly exercise, you'll benefit from carbs.

This brings me to a detour on crazy diets that make carbs the villain; there's no need to go on a low carb diet — 30% of calories from carbs or less — when your goal is fat loss. That is, unless you're 100% sedentary and do no form of exercise at all... which is a terrible idea for just about anyone.

Thousands of weight loss success stories have come from non-low carb diets, yet low carb diets are still engrained as the holy grail to fat loss in our society. Most people believe that carbohydrates get stored as fat, but that's not the case. Carbs can only be converted to fat (even a tiny amount) when in a caloric surplus.[6] There's even an entire book on using a high-carb, low fat diet (not low-carb) for fat loss. I won't get into it here, but you can read more about it at:

### *leanwithstyle.com/hcfl.*

Low carb diets do work, but there are negative health drawbacks. First of all, low carb diets are tough to maintain for long-term success. They are not sustainable for 90% of people.

They've been made popular through media such as fitness magazines, programs, and weight loss gurus in the mainstream media. These diets promise fast weight loss, but much of that weight is water weight and at times, muscle glycogen. Sure, the scale goes down, but for how long? No one asks for the "after-after" photo (e.g., how they look 1-2 years after their initial transformation photo).

There are more negative health drawbacks to low carb dieting, along with multiple studies that prove low carb diets are no better than a balanced macronutrient diet – but for now, let's resume our talk about carbs.

There are two types of carbohydrates:

- Complex carbs

- Simple carbs

Complex carbs come from complex starches such as those found in whole grains and vegetables. **I find complex carbs such as beans, sweet potatoes, and wheat bread to be the most satiating**. Simple carbs are foods such as white potatoes and white rice.

Which one is better for you depends on you and your testing. If you can get away with being in a caloric deficit and eating only simple carbs then go for it. However, if you start feeling a little hungry throughout the day, **try switching up your simple carbs with complex carbs.**

An easy example is to switch out your regular potatoes with sweet potatoes. It all comes down to testing and how satiated you feel during your weight loss journey. I personally go with a mix of simple carbs most of the time and still lose weight because it fits my macros and I feel full throughout the day. At the end of the day, both types of carbs get converted into glucose (AKA blood sugar) in the body.

With all that being said, pick carbs that you enjoy eating, adjust when necessary, and never fear carbs as they're necessary for fueling your body throughout your weight loss process. Here's a list of carbohydrates that I find nutritiously dense and filling:

- Potatoes

- Sweet Potatoes

- Lentils

- Oats

- White/brown rice

- Bread

- Fruits (e.g., apples, bananas, blueberries)

- Vegetables

Of course, some of these foods from the list intertwine with other lists from other macro categories. More on this soon.

## Dietary Fat

## (1 gram of fat = 9 calories)

Dietary fat has more than twice as many calories per gram as protein and carbohydrates.

Fats, like carbs, have also gotten a bad rap over the years. Back in the 90's, dietary fat was vilified for being "bad for you," which led to low fat diets.

VERY low-fat diets have negative drawbacks that can risk heart health, brain health, hormone imbalances, gut related problems, and much more. With that said, we also can't go overboard with dietary fats (the kind you eat) as they're the one macronutrient that's most **easily** converted into body fat.

There's research, however, that says a diet that's high-protein, high-carb, and low-fat results in the least amount of muscle loss, which is very important for dieting and body composition.[7][8]

For those reasons, I will recommend a diet that tends to lean towards the lower end of overall fat. The good news about dietary fat is that it provides flavor and promotes satiety in our meals. The trick is getting the right type of fats and the adequate amount of it in our diets.

Dietary fats can be broken down to two camps:

- Good fats

- Bad fats

Good fats consist of essential fatty acids (EFA) which are, as the name portrays, essential to the human body. These EFA's provide the body with hormone production and regulation, ensure proper adrenal and thyroid activity, and are crucial for the functionality of our brain and nervous system. The body can't survive without EFAs and can't produce them on its own. Therefore, we must get them from healthy food sources.

Here's a list of good fats:

- Olive oil

- Coconut oil

- Fish Oil

- Avocados

- Peanuts (peanut butter)

- Almonds

Of course, with the good comes some bad. Bad fats are man-made and are called trans-fats.

**Trans-fats** can be found in foods such as ice cream, cookies, cereals, fried foods, and lots of processed foods. Trans-fatty acids are responsible for raising the bad kind of cholesterol: LDL (low-density lipoproteins). Other side effects include heart disease, type 2 diabetes, and clogged arteries.

My experience with trans-fat, no surprises here, has been that they're not filling at all. For example, I love Circus Animal Cookies and they have trans-fat in their ingredients list. I would keep these cookies in my kitchen pantry... except I would "cheat" too often. When I used to log these cookies in the MFP app, I'd hit my macros, but I found myself feeling hungry the days I had a meal size worth of cookies.

So even if temptations such as treats that contain trans-fat can fit your macros, sometimes it's best to remove them from your kitchen as they don't positively help you move towards your overall goal.

In the age where food companies try their best to hide trans-fats in their nutrition labels, being nutrition-label-literate has never been more important.

Further investigating Circus Animal Cookies, their nutrition label's fine print states that 7 cookies (1 serving size) contain zero grams of trans fats (in 2015). That's zero trans fats in their cookies per serving. What gives? Here's where nutrition literacy comes into play.

These cookies actually do have trans-fat in them, but **FDA regulations state if the amount is less than 0.5 grams of trans-fat in a food serving, then the food manufacturer can label the product as zero grams of trans-fat.**[9]

Ask yourself, or someone you know, if they can stop at only one serving size of a favorite junk food snack. Most of the time, it's tough to stop — yet the trans-fat adds up. You'll know when a snack (usually processed foods) contains trans-fat, even when the brand doesn't have to label it, by checking the ingredients list.

Trans-fats ingredients start with the word "*hydrogenated.*" With our cookie example, the trans-fat disguised in the ingredients is called *Hydrogenated Palm Kernel Oil.*

Foods that often contain trans-fats are:

Tortilla chips

Cakes, cookies, and pastries

Deep fried foods (french fries and doughnuts come to mind)

The key takeaway here is that meal plans that contain trans-fat meals in significant portions will leave you un-satiated. Not to mention, there are negative health effects if trans-fats are overly consumed on a daily basis. But never eating these foods again and quitting cold turkey is **unrealistic.** Moderation is key when eating foods that come from the "bad fats" camp.

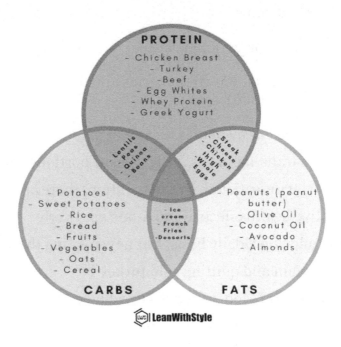

Now that we have gone over a list of foods and some notes for each macronutrient, I wanted to show you this image. As you can see, some foods intertwine with other macros. This list isn't final, but it should give you a good idea of what foods fall into what macro category.

# The Macronutrient and Calorie Relationship

Macronutrient recommendations, according to the Institutes of Medicine, calculated the following acceptable ranges[10]:

> 10-35% of calories should come from protein

> 45-65% of calories should come from carbohydrates

> 20-35% of calories should come from fats

Although these ranges are recommended, they're quite broad and not specific enough for someone who is aiming to lose body fat.

For the following examples, the format in which I'll be addressing macros are as follows:

### Protein / Carbs / Fat

*This format is often called "macro splits" or "macro ratios." It's a form of distributing your macros amongst your daily caloric intake by*

*percentages.*

The following macro ratios are common among the IIFYM and flexible dieting community:

1. 40% protein/40% carbs/20% fat

2. 30/40/30

3. 30/45/25

*Note: You can use any ratio you want and lose weight. These three ratios are those that I have seen work for most people. If you remain in a caloric deficit (obeying the law of energy balance) these ratios should work.*

Let's put macro ratios into perspective with an example.

We'll use a 200 lb. male, with maintenance calories of 3,000, for our example and use the **30/45/25** ratio.

Caloric Deficit (20% deficit) = 2,400 calories

# **30**/45/25

- 30% of calories from protein =
  0.30 x 2,400 = 720 calories

- Grams of protein per day =
  720 calories ÷ 4 grams/calories =
  **180 grams of protein per day**

## 30/**45**/25

- 45% of calories from carbs =
  0.45 x 2,400 = 1,080 calories

- Grams of carbs per day =
  1,080 calories ÷ 4 grams/calories =
  **270 grams of carbs per day**

## 30/45/**25**

- 25% of calories from dietary fat =
  0.25 x 2,400 = 600 calories

- Grams of fat per day =

  600 calories ÷ 9 grams/calories =

  **67 grams of fat per day**

**Total Macros and Calories:**

- 2400 Calories

- 180 g protein

- 270 g carbs

- 67 g fat

I have an IIFYM Calculator you can use in the course that will do all this math for you.

Smartphone apps like MFP can do these calculations for you; all you have to do is choose the macronutrient ratio that best suits you.

Your macro ratios, just like your caloric intake, are not set in stone. Adjust them when necessary (usually when what you're doing is not working). Remember that by tracking your macros, you also track calories which determines your weight loss or gain.

In the following image, my macro ratio is set to 30/ 40/ 30 but, on March 23rd, I felt like my body needed more carbs, so I didn't follow my macro ratio to the "T."

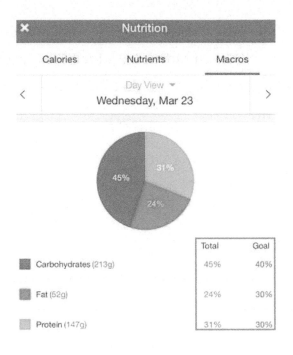

Protein is the most important macro to hit each day to preserve lean muscle tissue while losing fat. Your carbs and fats are debatable, but I like to keep my carbs relatively high and my fat no lower than 20-25%. **To ensure you're not gaining fat, make sure to stay within your daily calorie limit and you're golden; the weight will continue to come off**. At the same time, don't worry if you go over a little bit on your calories. Going over your caloric deficit by 50-100 calories won't impede your goal if it's not done every day.

Now that we know the math calculations, let's transition them to the MFP app.

## A Quick Introduction and User Guide to MyFitnessPal (MFP)

MFP is a very user-friendly smartphone application that's easy and quick to learn. However, there are a few important things to know beforehand.

When you create an account with MFP they will try and calculate your macros for you through a series of questions. I suggest **ignoring** their recommendations and setting up your macros with one of the ratios previously mentioned. After the MFP account setup, you can adjust your daily caloric intake and macro ratios. This can be done both on the app and on the MFP website. Taking the app as our reference, here is how to go about it.

- Tap on "More"
- Then "Goals"
- Under "Nutrition Goals," tap on "Calorie, Carbs, Protein, and Fat Goals"

From here, you'll be able to adjust your calories and macro ratios at any time. *I have more tutorials on how to do this step inside your free course.*

Once your macro ratio is set, MFP will distribute the calories for each macro based on your macro ratio percentages. Note that MFP "Premium" allows you to customize your daily macro settings with grams instead of percentages. You can opt for this option, but macro ratios based on percentages does the job.

**Logging Your Foods With The Phone Scanner Feature**

Logging your meals was a way to keep track of your meals nutrition details, and originally, flexible dieters would keep track of their daily macros in a notebook. These days we have MFP, and it's one of the best apps for logging in foods because of its awesome barcode scanner feature.

This feature lets you log your foods in an instant by simply scanning barcode labels. MFP then adds the content of the food towards your daily caloric and macro budget. This makes it easy to fill up your meal one, two, and so on for the day. And MFP will remember these meals for the next day, so you can easily add the previous day's meals without having to re-scan foods.

To use the scanner feature, follow these steps:

1. Open your MFP app and go to *Diary* > *Add Food* (under any meal).
2. The scan button will be at the top right of your screen (to the right of the search area).

3. Once the scanner launches, it should bring up your phone's camera.
4. Place the barcode of your specific food in front of your smartphone's camera and the scanner will capture the nutrition information once it's able to scan the barcode.

*Note: For this feature to work, you have to authorize MFP to access your camera (you should get prompted on your phone). If you haven't granted permission to MFP, you can do so under your phone's settings and not on the MFP app settings.*

I've created multiple tutorials for you to get started with MyFitnessPal.

These lessons include:

- How MyFitnessPal Works
- How to Setup MyFitnessPal on Your Phone
- How To Track Macros - Example 1

- How To Track Macros - Example 2

You can find these lessons in Part 2 of your IIFYM companion course (iifymbook.club).

# Chapter 4
# Getting Started with IIFYM

*"The greatest amount of wasted time is the time spent not getting started."*
*- Dawson Trotman*

If you've grasped the fundamentals in the prior chapters, you're ready to get started on your weight loss journey with flexible dieting at the wheel. IIFYM can seem a bit confusing when you're just starting out because you haven't put it into action yet. However, once you get started, you'll easily get the hang of it. As Radu Antoniu, creator of the ShredSmart Program, once said, *"When you look at foods, you'll feel like Neo inside the Matrix. All you see are numbers."*

In this chapter, we're going to cover more examples and an additional method of calculating your macros. Start calculating your own numbers if you haven't done so already; this way, you get comfortable with what you're learning.

## Calculating Your Macros For Cutting

"**Cutting**" refers to a weight loss phase whereas "**Bulking**" refers to a weight gain phase. We will use both terms in the following sections.

Recall, we need to start our calculations your TDEE or maintenance calories as we covered in Chapter 2. We'll use the same formula to calculate TDEE:

| Maintenance Calories (or TDEE) = | (*14 - 16*) x body weight (lbs) |
|---|---|

We'll use Mark, a 200 lb. male for this example, who is going on a "cut".

Mark knows that he leads a sedentary lifestyle and therefore chooses 14 as his multiplier which results in a TDEE of 2,800 calories (200 lbs. x 14 = 2,800). He wants to see results as quickly and as safe as possible, so he wants to be in an aggressive (but healthy) 25% caloric deficit. This places his daily intake at 2,100 calories per day (2,800 − 25% = 2,100) to lose weight.

Now that we have Mark's caloric deficit we can get his macro ratio in one of two ways.

1. The Macro Percentage method
2. The Macro Gram Per Pound Method

## The Macro Percentage Method

*We already covered this method in Chapter 3, so I'll keep this section brief.*

Mark can use any one of these three percentage ratios to calculate the grams required for each of the three macros (in the format: protein/carbohydrates/fats).

1. 40/40/20

2. 30/40/30

3. 30/45/25

Mark likes a fair amount of protein so he chooses the 40/40/20 ratio. Mark's macro distributions are as follows:

## Protein Intake

40% calories from proteins =

0.40 x 2,100 calories =

840 calories

Grams of protein per day =

840 calories ÷ 4 =

**210 grams of protein per day**

## **Carb Intake**

*(same calculation as protein – 40%)*

40% calories from carbs =

0.40 x 2,100 calories =

840 calories


Grams of carbs per day =

840 calories ÷ 4 =

**210 grams of carbs per day**


## **Fat Intake**

20% calories from fats =

0.20 x 2,100 calories =

420 calories


Grams of fats per day =

420 calories ÷ 9 =

**46.6 grams of fats per day**

Before we go over the totals, let's go over the other method.

## The Macro Gram Per Pound (g/lb.) Method

This is a common method you'll encounter at some point in your flexible dieting experience. It's a common method many in the flexible dieting community also use, so I decided to include it here. This method involves using standard values of grams that should be ingested for each macronutrient per pound of body weight.

The standards for the Gram Per Pound Method are as follows:

1.  **Protein**

    **0.82-1.2 Grams Of Protein Per Pound Of Body Weight.**

    If you don't enjoy protein in your diet as much, go with 0.82 as it's the lowest recommended protein intake recommended. If you tend to adhere to your diet better with more protein go with 1.2.

    1 gram is a perfect middle ground and has been the gold standard for decades.

2.  **Fats**

    **0.2 Grams of Fat Per Pound of Body Weight**

3. **Carbohydrates**

The rest of the calories are obtained from carbohydrates and fats.

Let's make sense of these gram per pound of body weight figures, shall we? We'll use Mark, who has a body weight of 200 lbs. with a 2,800 calorie TDEE and a caloric deficit intake of 2,100 calories, for this example.

## Protein Intake

1.2 x 200 lb. = **240 grams of protein per day**

Since 4 grams = 1 protein calorie, 960 calories will come from protein:

240 grams x 4 = 960 calories from protein.

*We'll use this number in a second for the calculation of your carb intake.*

## Fat Intake

0.2 x 200 lb. = **40 grams of fat per day**

Since 9 grams = 1 fat calorie, 360 calories will come from fat:

40 grams x 9 = 360 calories from fat.

*We'll use this number in a second for the calculation of your carb intake.*

## Carbohydrates Intake

2,100 calories – (960 calories from proteins + 360 calories from fats) = 780 calories

Knowing that 4 grams = 1 carb calorie:

780 calories ÷ 4 = **195 grams of carbs per day**

## Comparing the Percentage and the Gram Per Pound Method

Both methods are effective and common ways of calculating your macro intake in grams. Below is a table showing the comparison between the quantities obtained from both methods using Mark's example for cutting.

| Macro Intake | Percentage Method (40/40/20) | Gram/Pound Method |
|---|---|---|
| *Protein Intake* | 210g | 240g |
| *Carbohydrate Intake* | 210g | 195g |
| *Fats Intake* | 46.6g | 40g |
| *Total Calories* | 2100 | 2100 |

As you can see, the difference in macro portions obtained are minimal, yet the calories remain the same.

## Calculating Your Macros For Bulking

Although this book covers fat loss mostly, there will be a point in time when you eventually have to get out of a calorie deficit.

You cannot stay in one forever as this would cause many health problems. Therefore, once you've reached your weight loss goals, or after many months of cutting (whichever comes first), you want to bulk. "Many" months could be anything past 4 months where you are in a calorie deficit.

Sometimes a successful "Cut" can last 5 months, depending on how much weight you have to lose, so this time will vary for everyone. Just don't make the mistake of giving up too early and think "well, it's time to bulk I guess." If you're not seeing results from your diet or hitting weight loss plateaus, we will go over what to do soon.

Lastly, before we get to your bulking macros and calories, do NOT think that bulking means you get to eat everything under the proverbial sun. **You are only increasing calories and that is IT.**

It is not an excuse to eat whatever you want. You are simply putting yourself in a small surplus (5-10%) to maximize muscle growth while minimizing fat gain. With all that being said about bulking, let's turn back to our example with Mark.

We are going to use Mark this time, but we are going to tweak his "stats" to make it more sensible for him to bulk.

Let's say, with the previous calculations, he lost 20 lbs. and now weighs 180 lbs. He is no longer sedentary. In fact, with his new physique, he is now more active (e.g., trains 4-6 times per week for 1-2 hours each session).

His new maintenance calories, based on multiplying his new body weight in lbs. by 15.5 are:

**180 x 15.5 = 2790 Maintenance Calories**

*Remember, he is more active now, so we no longer use 14. We don't use the high end (16) because he isn't super active though either.*

Now that we have Mark's new maintenance calories of 2790, **we must add calories to put Mark in a caloric surplus.**

To make sure Mark doesn't gain weight back too quickly, we want to put him in a small 5-10% surplus (**Note**: *after you calculate your calories, you would follow the macro calculation steps we did previously*):

**2790 x .05 = 140 calories**

**2790 x .10 = 279 calories**

*(I calculated both options to show you the difference between a 5-10% surplus).*

Now, we add the calories from the above calculations to his maintenance calories.

**2790 + 140 = 2930 calories (+5% surplus)**

**2790 +279 = 3069 calories (+10% surplus)**

If I were coaching Mark, I would recommend he start out at a 5% surplus and see how his body responds for the first 2 weeks. If he is not gaining at least 0.5-1 pound per week, he would then increase to the 10% surplus option and check his progress again after 2 weeks.

**Again, these formulas don't mean anything if you don't check your progress.** Make sure you do that, so you don't put weight back on too quickly. Inevitably, you will see some fat gain due to the law of energy balance. This is expected. Don't worry about this. **Think of Cutting and Bulking as a "3 steps forward, 1 step back," method:**

- You cut down to a weight you are happy with (let's say from 200 lbs. to 180 lbs.).

- You bulk up to a weight that is lower than your previous starting weight (187-190 lbs.). You look better than before because you put on muscle (hopefully) through being in a surplus and working out.

- You cut again, but this time, you lose more weight that before (175lbs) while holding on to most of your muscle, if not all.

- You bulk again, this time only putting a few more pounds (182 lbs.), mostly coming from muscle.

- Rinse and repeat.

Now this is how it's SUPPOSED to look, but we are not perfect. Things will happen and it will take some trial and error. Don't be hard on yourself if your cutting and bulking attempts don't look this the first time around.

It's only a goal to strive towards.

## Your Macro Calculations

*Note: If you want to see more macro calculation examples, I've included some in part 3 of your bonus companion course (iifymbook.club).*

Now it's your turn. Use this page to help calculate your macros. Below I've entered the fields you need to input in order to calculate your macros using the Percentage method.

## Step 1: Find Your Maintenance Calories (TDEE) :

| | | |
|---|---|---|
| 14 - 16 x B.W. = | ____ x ____ lb. = | _____ Maintenance Calories (TDEE) |

## Step 2: Find Your Caloric Deficit:

| | | |
|---|---|---|
| TDEE – (20% OR 25%) = | ____ - (20% OR 25%) = | _____ Calories For Weight Loss |

*Note: for macro calculations choose between the following macro ratio (protein/carbs/fat):*

- 40/40/20

- 30/40/30

- 30/45/25

I'll use the rate 30/40/30 for the fill-in-the blank template below, but feel free to swap those numbers out. Also, your "caloric deficit" is the number you calculated from step 2.

### Step 3: Find Your Protein Macros (30%):

| = 0.30 x caloric deficit | = (0.30 x _____) ÷ 4 = | _____ Grams of Protein Per Day |
|---|---|---|
| | | |

### Step 4: Find Your Carb Macros (40%):

| = 0.40 x caloric deficit | = (0.40 x _____) ÷ 4 = | _____ Grams of Carbs Per Day |
|---|---|---|
| | | |

## Step 5: Find Your Fat Macros (30%):

| = 0.30 x caloric deficit | = (0.30 x _____) ÷ 9 = | _____ Grams of Fat Per Day |
|---|---|---|
| | | |

Although you can have my included calculator (found in your course) or MyFitnessPal do this for you, **there's a value in doing the calculation by hand** at least a couple times so you really understand your starting point and nutritional numbers. Doing this will help you adjust your deficit and macros down the road if you hit a plateau or want to change your macro ratios.

# Chapter 5
# Meal Planning Success

*"Failing to plan is planning to fail." – Jim Rohn*

After you've calculated your macros, the next step is to make your IIFYM meal plan. Having a meal plan is not required, but it is recommended. Meal planning gives you an understanding of your caloric consumption and makes it easier for you to stay within your macronutrient limits.

A common challenge for IIFYM beginners is adapting to tracking meals, measuring quantities with a food scale and things related of this nature. This usually stems from the "I'll wing it" approach to IIFYM. Although it can be done, it's not good practice when starting out. **To have the most success with IIFYM for weight loss, follow the guidelines in this chapter for the first two months.** Track everything. Then, you can ease off a bit.

## Kitchen Tools For Measuring Your Macros

Not all of your foods are going to come with the exact serving sizes you want to eat. You'll have to measure some foods first before you can add them to your MFP app. A good example of this is olive oil. A serving size is 1 tablespoon and typically 119 calories with 14 grams of fat. You might be in a position where a serving size of olive oil can put you over your fat macros by a few grams (which in terms of the fat macro can add up fast).

Instead, half a serving size of olive oil would fit perfectly within your macros. In this case, you'll use a 0.5 tablespoon and adjust the serving size on your MFP app accordingly. Situations like this are frequent and you're bound to come across them with volume and weighted serving sizes.

Here's the list of required tools to have in your kitchen to accurately account for different macros, volumes, and weight:

1.  Measuring Cups

2. Measuring Tablespoons
3. A Digital Food Scale
4. MyFitnessPal App, which is available for iOS and Android

## A Step By Step Guide To Creating Your Meal Plan

The 10 questions below don't have to be answered right away. They are just questions to consider when following the steps to create your meal plan, and they're some of the questions I ask clients who want a meal plan.

1. What time do you wake up?

2. What time do you go to bed?

3. What time do you work out?

4. How many times per week do you exercise?

5. Do you work out fasted?

6. What foods do you love?

7. What foods do you dislike/hate?

8. What sauces do you use?

9. Will protein powder supplements contribute to your protein intake?

10. What meal would you want to be the biggest? Breakfast, lunch, or dinner?

Again, no need to answer these questions right now, but they're questions to consider to create the optimal meal plan for you.

## Step 1 – List Your Foods

Start by listing the foods you want included in your daily meal plan. Either write down your food list or make a digital list (in Excel or Google Sheets). Make sure to include the quantities of each macro and the calories it contains in side-by-side columns along with the serving size. Try out the MFP scanner feature to add foods that are already in your kitchen! You can also go to MFP's food database for more nutritional information on foods you can't find original barcodes or nutritional information for.

Doing this step will help you include your favorite carbs, proteins, and fats when you begin to form your meals.

Here's an example of how you would do this:

| Protein Sources | Calories per Serving | Protein (Grams) | Carbs (Grams) | Fat (Grams) |
| --- | --- | --- | --- | --- |
| Chicken Breast (4 oz) | 120 | 26 | 0 | 1 |
| 96% Fat Free Ground Beef (4 oz) | 150 | 24 | 0 | 5 |
| 99% Fat Free Ground Turkey (4 oz) | 120 | 28 | 0 | 1 |
| Flank Steak (4 oz) | 180 | 24 | 0 | 9 |
| Legion Protein Powder (29 grams) | 100 | 22 | 3 | 0 |
| Kodiak Cakes Pancake Mix (53 grams) | 190 | 14 | 30 | 2 |

| Carb Sources | Calories per Serving | Protein (Grams) | Carbs (Grams) | Fat (Grams) |
| --- | --- | --- | --- | --- |
| Red Potatoes (4 oz) | 84 | 2 | 20 | 0 |
| Sweet Potatoes (4 oz) | 97 | 2 | 23 | 0 |
| Brown Rice (100 grams) | 111 | 3 | 23 | 1 |
| Lentils (100 grams) | 116 | 9 | 20 | 0 |

| Fat Sources | Calories per Serving | Protein (Grams) | Carbs (Grams) | Fat (Grams) |
| --- | --- | --- | --- | --- |
| Avocado Oil (1 tbsp) | 124 | 0 | 0 | 14 |
| Organic PB Fit (16 grams) | 70 | 8 | 5 | 2 |
| Almonds (1 oz) | 160 | 6 | 6 | 14 |

I've left a couple things out like veggies, sauces, and fruit, but the spreadsheet above is to give you an idea of this step.

## Step 2 – Creating Your Meals

Once you've filled out your favorite foods for each macro category, start making your meals the same day or the next day so you can get used to it. This way, after a few days of your meal plan you'll know if you're satisfied with it or not.

When creating a meal, I like to follow the Chipotle (a Mexican grill in the U.S.) structure. For example, their burrito bowls are a great **meal template to follow**. First, they have you pick your carbs (brown or white rice). Then your protein (chicken, steak, etc.). Then veggies (lettuce or fajita vegetables). Then your salsas (mild, medium or hot). Finally, you add your fats (cheese or guac) and that's it.

It's simple and something you should keep in mind when creating your meal plan. You don't have to follow everything exactly like Chipotle does, but it's a good template to follow for at least one of your meals.

## An Example Meal Plan

Here's what a meal plan would look like for a 200 lb. male. I used the new IIFYM calculator (found in the free companion course) to "configure" the calories and macros. To create this, I pulled foods from each macro category (on the list that I created in step 1) and grouped them into meals that I believed to be filling and satisfying, along with some of my favorites.

## Pre-Workout Snack (Break-Fast)

| Food | How Much | Calories | Carbs | Fat | Protein |
|---|---|---|---|---|---|
| Whey Protein (see notes) | 45 g | 182 | 3 | 2 | 33 |
| Banana | 100 g | 89 | 29 | 9 | 1 |
| Almond Milk | 240 mL | 30 | 0 | 3 | 1 |
| **TOTAL** | | **301** | **23** | **5** | **35** |

 **Workout (taken with Legion Pulse Before and Recharge/ Creatine After)**

## Post-Workout Meal

| | Food | How Much | Calories | Carbs | Fat | Protein |
|---|---|---|---|---|---|---|
| (Part1) | Olive Oil | .5 tbsp | 60 | 0 | 7 | 0 |
| | Chicken Breast (raw weight) | 10 oz | 300 | 0 | 3 | 65 |
| | Sweet Potato (uncooked weight) | 250 g | 215 | 50 | 0 | 4 |
| (Part2) | Olive Oil | .5 tbsp | 60 | 0 | 7 | 0 |
| | Egg Whites | 276 g | 150 | 0 | 0 | 30 |
| | Mushrooms | 30 g | 7 | 1 | 0 | 1 |
| | Onions | 30 g | 12 | 3 | 0 | 0 |
| | Bell Peppers | 50 g | 10 | 2 | 0 | 0 |
| | Tomatoes | 30 g | 5 | 1 | 0 | 0 |
| | **TOTAL** | | **819** | **57** | **17** | **100** |

LEAN WITH STYLE

*Part 1 of 2*

## Dinner (aka. FEAST)

| | Food | How Much | Calories | Carbs | Fat | Protein |
|---|---|---|---|---|---|---|
| (Part1) | Kodiak Cake Chocolate Chip Pancakes | 106 g | 400 | 60 | 6 | 28 |
| | Whey Protein (see notes) | 15 g | 60 | 1 | 1 | 11 |
| | Sugar Free Syrup | 60 mL | 15 | 6 | 0 | 0 |
| (Part2) | Chobani Greek Yogurt | 255 g | 195 | 24 | 0 | 21 |
| | Peanut Butter | 32 g | 190 | 6 | 16 | 7 |
| | Banana | 115 g | 102 | 23 | 0 | 1 |
| | Whey Protein | 15 g | 60 | 1 | 1 | 11 |
| | TOTAL | | 1022 | 121 | 24 | 79 |

| | | | | | |
|---|---|---|---|---|---|
| Daily Total | 2143 | 201 | 46 | 216 |
| Goal For Day | 2120 | 213 | 47 | 213 |
| | | 40% Carbs | 20% Fat | 40% Protein |

*Part 2 of 2*

As you can see in the last couple rows, the macro goals weren't met to the gram, however, that's not a big deal and minuscule in the grand scheme of things as this individual is only 23 calories over his goal. Furthermore, if you feel like having a bit more carbs, then do it — just make sure to remove some macros from your daily fat goal. As long as you're within +/- 50 (100 tops) calories of your calorie goals, it shouldn't impede your progress. Just make sure you're tracking everything to see what delays or improves your progress.

**Some Notes on the Example Meal Plan**

- **Produce/Veggies** — I used MFP to calculate these calories and macros, specifically the USDA version (if you use the food search method in MFP). Your calories and macros may vary slightly.
- **Intermittent Fasting (IF)** – Whether you follow IF or not, you can still follow this meal plan. If you DO follow IF, then your first meal is the one that breaks your

fast. Your fasting window can be whatever you want. Watch the video in the course to learn more about IF.

- **Kodiak Cakes** – I have been eating Kodiak Cakes for the past 3 years and I don't plan on stopping anytime soon. I suggest trying them out. They are packed with protein and delicious. You can usually find them for bulk on Amazon or Costco or a similar store.

- **Sauces, Seasonings, and Sweeteners** – You may use sweeteners like stevia and vanilla extract if you wish. Sauces are fine too (i.e., bbq sauce, teriyaki sauce, ranch, etc.) however, take into account their calories and macros as they are usually packed with them. Also, if you want some nice zero calories syrups, Walden Farms has some good ones (i.e., chocolate, blueberry, and regular syrup). Lastly, seasonings are fine to use and not necessary to track unless your seasoning has a substantial amount of calories (i.e., more than 30 calories per serving).

- **Supplements** – I've written an entire article on what the best supplements for cutting are (bit.ly/best_cs). Below are some notes on each that I use in the meal plan.

- **Whey Protein** – You may use any protein brand you like; however, I use Legion WHEY+ Protein, specifically, their Cinnamon Cereal flavor because it's so damn delicious. I'd also recommend the Optimum Nutrition Gold Standard Whey Protein brand as well. It's not as tasty as Legion's but it is a bit cheaper.

- **Pre-Workout** – I use Legion Pulse and I suggest you do too. It's the best pre-workout I've ever had and LabDoor ranks it #1 in terms of quality and purity amongst all the pre-workout supplements they have ever tested, which is in the hundreds.

- **Creatine** – I always take creating while cutting. It helps with recovery and performance in the gym. I use the one from Optimum Nutrition because it's cheap and high-quality. You can just mix it in with water or any protein shake, etc.

Also note that this is just a **sample meal plan** and will not work for everyone or fill everyone's satisfaction. You might like to have your largest meal at night or workout fasted. You might not like to use supplements and may prefer actual food instead. Again, it's your meal plan, so make it fit your needs, your schedule, **and ultimately, make sure it fits your macros.**

*If you want to download the macro spreadsheet and other **sample meal plans**, you can find more in your bonus companion course.*

## Step 3 – Adjust Your Meal Plan

Don't be surprised if you have to adjust your meal plan during the first week. Explore your meal options with different foods until you get meal combinations that you are satisfied with. After a week or two, you'll see what meals you can, and can't, live without.

## FAQ's For Meal Planning And IIFYM In General

### *FAQ 1: What Is The Best Time To Eat And How Often?*

The only key is that you stick to your daily macro requirements, whether you choose to have a huge breakfast or a huge lunch! **Note:** there are some scientific recommendations if you work out a lot — particularly for those who do weight training.

Research shows that 30-50g of carbohydrates is recommended pre-workout.[11]

Research has also shown that when you are doing plenty of weightlifting workouts, eating some protein before your workout sessions is a sure way to build muscle and subsequently get stronger over time.[12] However, post-workout protein is more important than pre-workout protein. **The recommended quantities here are around 30-40g of protein-rich foods just before and after your workout.**

When it comes to frequency of your meals, again, it is all up to your personal preferences whether you will stick to three meals or have seven meals in a day. Provided you manage your energy levels and balance out your macronutrients as required, the frequency of meals and the timings do not have much effect on your weight loss results.

However, if you have pre-existing health conditions such as diabetes, for example, which require you to eat often, you have to ensure you plan your meals accordingly and stick to your limits to avoid overindulging.

### FAQ 2: Other Than Pre- And Post-Workout Meals, When Should I Eat My Meals?

You should eat whenever works best for you. It honestly depends on your schedule. There is no difference when you eat your meals in the large, weekly view of things.

### FAQ 3 : Should I Eat Differently On Days That I Don't Lift Or Do Cardio?

You shouldn't change a thing. Stick to your meal plan and make sure you're hitting your macros. Since you're already in a deficit, weight loss should still occur. If you remember, we took your maintenance calories (TDEE) and subtracted 25% from it. On the days you don't lift or do cardio, you might not be in a 25% deficit, but you're in a deficit nonetheless. There are things such as calorie-cycling on training and rest days, however, for weight loss, I've found that keeping a consistent calorie deficit day to day works best.

### FAQ 4: Should I Log My Meal Before Or After Eating It?

When I started out, I used to eat all day while estimating whether I was within my limits, then log in all the random things I ate at the end of the day. The problem with that approach was that being accurate became harder and harder over time. Sometimes you find that you ate all your carbs during the day and now your dinner has to be 3g of fat and 20g of protein! The solution to avoiding this is the MFP app on your phone, considering that you have your phone everywhere you go.  Simply put: *Log It Before You Eat It*!

This is a very simple rule to follow, but it will make all the difference! If you want to eat something, log it first. This will ensure that you are 100% efficient and successful when it comes to hitting your macro limits.

Ideally, planning your day beforehand and logging your day in advance is the best scenario. However, sometimes you want a little freedom and spontaneity with your meals; just ensure you remain within your calorie limits.

## FAQ 5: What Are The Recommended Foods For Flexible Dieting?

As mentioned above, IIFYM is loved for its flexibility in choice. Ideally, you can eat whatever it is you want and love provided it fits your macros. However, **just because you can does not mean you should** live on junk! Processed foods tend to have their limitations especially when it comes to fiber content, excessive fats, and limited vitamin and mineral content. Therefore, for optimal functioning of your body, you have to balance junk with foods that have nutrients that you will most definitely not get from Pop-Tarts, ice cream, and your assortment of candy.

With that in mind, at least 80% of your daily caloric intake should be derived from nutritious meals which are unprocessed. Some examples of tasty, nutritious foods that you can opt for include:

- Peanuts, peas, lentils, eggs, yogurt, cashews, almonds, and beans like pinto, navy, black, kidney, and garbanzo.

- Seeds like sunflower, quinoa, sesame, pumpkin, and flax.

- Avocados, bananas, berries, mushrooms, and Brussels sprouts

- Greens like spinach, broccoli, kales, mustard greens, collard greens, and chard.

- Sweet potatoes, baked potatoes, whole grains like brown rice, wheat, barley, and oats.

- Chicken, turkey, lamb, tuna, shrimp, lean beef, salmon, scallops, and halibut.

- The list could go on and on.

At your local grocery store, you'll always find new foods that fit your macros perfectly.

For example, I have pancakes every morning. Specifically, Kodiak Cakes. They have great macros (you can see in the meal plan example earlier in the chapter) and are another reason why IIFYM is awesome. If you have a certain food that you love but the macros aren't exactly great, there's usually an alternative you can find.

### FAQ 6: What Foods Should I Avoid?

Watch out for super calorie-rich foods. These are foods that sneak up on you calorie wise. Before starting my IIFYM diet, I had almost no idea how many calories some of the things I loved carried.

I recommend completely avoiding caloric beverages, especially soda. One large Coke can be filled with hundreds of calories and barely fill you up; not to mention all the other ingredients inside it. Another example we can look at is beer. An occasional beer when you get to the house from a stressful day is not too foreign. However, a can of beer or even a single glass can have up to 100-200 calories.

If you love macadamia nuts, a small pack of 100g has well over 600 calories! This is the same case for some foods like peanut butter, dried fruit, coffee creamer, dark chocolate, dairy products, granola bars, hummus, salad dressing, trail mix and frozen yogurt; the list is endless.

Another interesting one is shots of vodka where a single shot carries around 125 nutrient-less calories (not to mention the chaser). This is the equivalent of chugging a medium Dunkin' cappuccino! So next time you are planning for a night out, **remember to plan ahead and have enough calories left for your vodka or beers.**

### *FAQ 7: How Big Should My Meals Be?*

This all depends on how many calories you have to deal with.  If you have 2000 calories, for example, your meals should be either evenly dispersed (calorie wise) or dispersed in a way that compliments your style of eating.

If you want to evenly disperse your meals, it would look something like this:

- Meal 1: 500 calories

- Meal 2: 500 calories

- Meal 3: 500 calories

- Meal 4: 500 calories

If you want to distribute your calories in a way that compliments your style of eating (let's say you like having a big lunch), it would look something like this:

- Meal 1: 350 calories

- Meal 2: 1000 calories

- Meal 3: 650 calories

It all honestly depends on your style of eating. Personally, I like the second method better since I like big meals.

### FAQ 8: What If I Get Hungry?

It's going to happen. After all, you're feeding your body less and less. However, I've found that the best way to combat this is simply adding some volume to your meals to create the "full" feeling.

This is a very simple trick, but it works! You can do this in two main ways:

1. Substitute very calorie-rich foods with foods that are more nutrient-dense (e.g., sweet potatoes instead of white bread for lunch).

2. Mixing in vegetables with your carbs and protein meals. For example, you could cut up some mushrooms, bell peppers, tomatoes, and spinach and mix it in with your meat or carbs. The vegetables are low in calories but high in volume, thus creating a satiating effect. For example, a bowl-full of spinach is 20 calories. That's a lot of spinach!

Feel free to get as innovative as possible with your meals since that is the whole essence of IIFYM.

### FAQ 9: What Happens If I Miss My Calorie/Macro Target?

Of course, rule number one of IIFYM fight club is stick to your macro targets :)

However, what happens if you end up missing your targets? Unlike other diets, missing the mark once or twice is not the end of your weight loss journey, and it will not have a big effect on your body composition goals in the grand scheme of things.

The advantage of being in a 20-25% deficit of your maintenance calories is that even if you exceed your limit by a little (100-150 calories), you are still below your maintenance calorie levels and therefore will not be gaining any extra weight. But take extra care not to end up being in a surplus, since this would now present a whole new problem.

A caloric surplus means you are giving your body more energy (calories) than it needs and this could very well end up being a recipe for disaster!

If you hit surplus, do not cut your diet immensely the next day. Remember that the aim of IIFYM is to help with weight loss but do so responsibly to avert from starvation. Your maximum food deficit should not be higher than 25%.

This means that if your maintenance is 3,000 calories, your maximum deficit can be:

$$25\% \text{ (maximum deficit)} \times 3{,}000 \text{ (maintenance calories)} = 750 \text{ calories}$$
$$3000 - 750 = 2250 \text{ calories}$$

Your smallest daily target should, therefore, be 2250 calories. All in all, do not get down on yourself too much if you miss your mark occasionally — especially when starting out. Learn from your mistakes and remember that your diet will only be effective if you stick to it as much as possible.

### *FAQ 10: Can I Drink Alcohol?*

Of course you can, just in moderation. Alcohol has its own macronutrient content —carbs — thus, you should track accordingly. For example, if you know you're going out drinking, leave some room for alcohol and remove some carbs from your meals throughout the day. In a later chapter, I go over more specific tips on how to eat "dirty" foods or drinks without losing your sanity.

### *FAQ 11: What Does An Example Day Look Like For You?*

I follow intermittent fasting when dieting so I save up my calories for a specific period from 2-10pm. It looks like this:

- *2pm*
  **Small Pre-Workout Meal:** This meal is usually less than 500 calories and follows rules previously mentioned (i.e., 30-40g protein).

- *5pm*
  **Post-Workout Meal:** This meal is usually 700-1000 calories and my biggest meal of the day.

- *9pm*
  **Meal 3:** This meal is usually a "tastier" meal, but still high in protein and carbs. For the past couple of months, this has usually been Kodiak Cakes (pancakes at night... I know).

- *10pm*
  **Meal 4:** I usually choose some treat like

Halo Top or Greek yogurt with peanut butter.

If you want to see another example, there's a 'full day of eating video' found in your companion course.

### FAQ 12: What About Cheat Days?

Cheat "Days" are not allowed. **One cheat day could set you back a whole week. Seriously.** Especially if you over do it. Instead, have a cheat **meal** or a "refeed" day. Let's go over what each is briefly and why they're necessary.

A cheat meal is exactly what it says. You have one meal of whatever you'd like once a week. No need to track the calories or macros for it; just have something you're craving.

A refeed day is where you increase the amount of carbohydrates you eat by 100-150 grams (400-600 calories) once a week.

We follow one of the choices above because of one specific hormone: leptin. Leptin is responsible for multiple functions within the body, however, the one we're worried about is your metabolism. When you're in a caloric deficit and trying to lose weight, your leptin levels begin to drop.[13] When this happens, your metabolism begins to slow down, thus making it harder to lose weight despite being in a deficit.

Enter refeed days or cheat meals. Eating carbs is one way to increase leptin levels. Refeed days are specifically designed to increase carbs dramatically, thus increasing leptin levels for a bit. Cheat meals usually contain a lot of carbohydrates; however, this isn't always the case. Sometimes a cheat meal can contain lots of fat and very little protein or carbs. **I don't recommend this.** If you go the cheat meal route, make sure it's a high carb meal, if possible.

Personally, I prefer refeed days because I can spread out the carbs more throughout the day, however, sometimes, unexpected events happen, and I'll just decide to have my cheat meal then.

## Quick Note on Meal Prepping

The following are tips for meal *prepping,* not
meal planning. If you have a busy schedule and
have little to no time to cook, meal prepping is
efficient and can save you a lot of time.

### *Tip 1 – Plan Two Dedicated Meal Prep Days*

Pick two days out of the week to prep your meals
after you've chosen what foods you want to eat.
For example, Sunday and Wednesday can be meal
prep days. On Sunday, you would take 1-3 hours
to cook a big amount of your protein and carbs of
choice and spread them out into the containers.
Depending on however many meals you plan on
having for each day, you would make enough
meals to last you till Wednesday. If you're cooking
a lot of protein on your meal prep day, for
example chicken, weigh your chicken serving size
uncooked. This is the way you'll track most meats
with MFP.

The reason I recommend meal prepping until

Wednesday and not for the whole week is that food doesn't taste as good if it's in the fridge for more than three days... and veggies usually start to have a foul odor. On Wednesday I repeat the process and prep my meals up until Friday.

*Don't forget to measure your foods to get accurate calories and macros for your meals. If you eat the same meals every day, you can "create" these meals in MFP and track them with 1-2 buttons, making it super convenient.*

I only meal prep up to Friday because I like to cook different meals on weekends or go out to eat with friends or family. Meal prepping isn't for everyone, but if it helps you stick to your meal plan, I recommend it.

### Tip 2 – Mix Up Your Meals When Needed

If need be, switch meals up so that your meals don't become boring. Some people do better eating the same thing every day as long as it fits their macros — especially if they're eating what they like. However, in my case, I don't particularly enjoy eating the same proteins every day for weeks.

Instead, what I like to do is eat one source of protein for a given week and then change the source. For example, if for the first week all my meals protein came from chicken breast, the next week would all come from ground turkey. The following week would be ground beef and then back to chicken breast and so on.

Mixing it up like this will not only get you a variety of nutrients and protein, but also keep your meals from being un-exciting. If you like how your meals are, then don't change a thing. Again, some people can eat the same thing every day and that's perfectly fine!

### *Tip 3 – Give Yourself An Unscheduled Meal*

If you can, leave one meal for the day that is not prepped. For example, if you eat 4 meals per day, one of those meals can be cooked fresh. This is a good strategy for people who love and can't be without breakfast food (eggs, bacon, etc.). However, you can also save the last meal of the day for a treat. Make that last, un-prepped meal something that you look forward to every day. I recommend the ice cream brand *Halo Top* because the macros on it are amazing (low fat and high protein) and a whole pint is roughly 320 calories, depending on which flavor you get.

All in all, IIFYM is not the easiest dietary concept out there, but at the same time, it's not rocket science either. You simply must give yourself time to learn, adjust your lifestyle, and in no time the results will start to become evident. IIFYM is the most accurate dieting concept I have come across to date, and I can honestly attribute all my weight loss success to it!

# Chapter 6
# The IIFYM Journey

*"You don't have to be great to get started, but you have to get started to be great."*
*– Ralf W. Emerson*

If It Fits Your Macros is and will continue to be, a popular protocol for proper dieting. After a week or so of putting flexible dieting to practice, you'll realize that it's a style of eating that you can potentially carry with you for the rest of your life. You can use it to whether your goal is to lose, gain, or maintain weight, with flexibility built for healthy weight management.

I remember when I first started IIFYM during a weight loss phase. **It wasn't until I started tracking macros that I started seeing results.** The results will come once you start putting the knowledge you gain from this book to action. If you're new to IIFYM, and you're in a "paralysis analysis phase," don't sweat it. You got this!

Take baby steps by first calculating your caloric deficit and then your macros. Next, download the MyFitnessPal (MFP) app on your phone (or a similar app that can track calories and macros). My challenge to you is to have a successful day of tracking your macros following what's taught in this book, then try a week of IIFYM. Eventually it'll become second nature and you'll minimize the amount of times you have to check in with MFP.

**The Road Ahead**

As the weeks progress, you may notice that weight loss starts to get progressively challenging. Weight loss, like any other goal, gets tough towards the end stages. It doesn't help that our bodies are genetically wired to "hold on to" as many fat stores as it can when we're a caloric deficit. It's just how we're genetically wired. The two pounds a week we lost the first weeks eventually becomes one pound a week because your body is losing energy (fat stores) it once had as a reserve. The body freaks out and works against us. Be aware of this towards the "end game" of your weight loss journey.

In the words of Steven Pressfield from his book *The War of Art*, "*The danger is greatest when the finish line is in sight. At this point, Resistance knows we're about to beat it. It hits the panic button. It marshals one last assault and slams us with everything it's got.*"

If you track your IIFYM weight loss journey, you'll realize that fluctuation is also part of the game. In the following pages, for instance, there's a screenshot of my weight loss fluctuations over the last few months. **I hope I'm not the bearer of bad news, but you must know that your weight loss phase won't be linear.** It'll be a bit messy and will have peaks and valleys when you track your weight.

Let's go over why fluctuations happen and how to adjust when the inevitable weight loss plateau occurs.

## Understanding the Weight Loss Plateau

You see, weight loss can be funny. You're doing everything right. You're hitting your macros. You're doing your cardio. You're lifting heavy. And you drop maybe half a pound by the end of the week. Heck, maybe you even gain a pound! Don't panic. There are a lot of reasons the scale may not be going down.

When people don't see the scale going down every single day, they panic and start doing extra work. They start doing a lot more cardio and begin subtracting hundreds of calories, or they just give up. Do NOT take this approach. First, let's diagnose the problem.

## Your Sodium and Potassium Intake

Your salt intake could be a reason why the scale isn't moving in the direction you'd like. When you overeat salt, your body holds onto it, and this causes water retention and causes you to be "bloated."

Note: Bloating can be caused by other factors as well.

Therefore, some micronutrient tracking can be beneficial. Potassium has the opposite effect of sodium. **Whereas salt holds onto the water, potassium flushes it out**. The daily recommended sodium intake is about 2.3 grams or 2300 mg. (If you sweat a lot, your intake may be a bit higher.)

In MFP, under the "nutrients" tab in your diary, you can see your sodium and potassium content for the day. The daily recommended potassium intake is about 4.7 grams a day or 4700 mg.

To avoid sodium and potassium imbalances, make sure to avoid most canned/packaged foods as well as deli meats. They're all usually high in sodium.

**Other foods that are usually high in sodium:**

- Sauces and salad dressings

- Cheese

- Fast foods

**Foods that are high in potassium are:**

- Salmon

- Mushrooms

- Yogurt

- Beans

- Potatoes

- Bananas

I'm not saying you should track sodium and potassium like you would your regular macros (protein, fat, and carbs). I just want you to be aware of it and check nutrition labels when possible.

Also, a quick note on water. **I recommend you have at least a gallon of water a day**, which should be enough for most people. However, some of us are more active than others and sweat more than others, so a gallon may not be enough. A gallon of water for someone who is sedentary compared to someone who does construction every day is not going to be equivalent. **Therefore, to judge your water needs, make sure to have 4-5 clear urinations each day.**

### "Hidden" Calories

Another reason you may not be losing weight is that you aren't aware of "hidden" calories or you're just not tracking them in MFP. New dieters usually deal with this. These are calorics you aren't aware of, such as dressings, sauces, oil, etc. Make sure to count the amount of oil you use when cooking, for example. **Two tablespoons of olive oil range from 200-240 calories!**

What about that ranch or BBQ sauce? That could be another 200 calories right there. Plus, sauces like BBQ sauce are packed with sodium. Another example is coffee. I love drinking black coffee every morning, and so do a lot of people. But most people put cream in their coffee which can be an additional 80-150 calories. **Yes, these little calories add up.**

If you don't take into account the "little" things, then your fat loss journey will take much longer. You don't want that. I know it may seem a little tedious to account for your oil and your ketchup, but hidden calories are very real and could be the reason that your weight loss is stalling.

If you typically don't add sauces or dressings, then you don't necessarily have to track small things like ketchup. Just be AWARE of it.

**Your Activity Levels**

You can also just be overestimating how active you are. If you sit at home all day and the only activity you have is going to the gym, but you said you were lightly active, your calorie deficit may be too small.

There are two solutions to this:

## 1. Decrease calories (from carbohydrates)

That is, subtract 100 calories (25g of carbs) from your diet. Before you do this, try option 2:

## 2. Move more.

I always recommend moving more before decreasing calories. By move more, I mean just getting out and being more active:

- Walk to the gym.

- Go for a walk with your dog (or by yourself) every day.

- Go on hikes every weekend.

- Add an extra cardio session.

- Just be more active.

I say this because my brother and I work from home a lot.

We're pretty much at our computers 80% of the day (we're going to switch this soon and be more active), so we invested in a standing desk.

**Always try moving more before decreasing calories**. It doesn't hurt to get out more often.

**What if:**

- Your sodium and potassium levels are normal,

- You're doing your cardio and weights and being more active,

- You're aware of hidden calories and,

- You're hitting your macros...

And the scale still isn't going down? Don't give up just yet.

Know that the scale isn't the best measurement for success in your weight — and especially fat — loss journey. There are better and more accurate ways to check your fat loss status.

Do the following every day:

## 1. Weigh yourself every morning after you've used the bathroom.

Every morning, go number 2 (if you can) and then weigh yourself. Then, once you've weighed yourself and the scale hasn't gone down, don't freak out just yet.

Keep track of your daily weigh-ins in a notebook or on MFP. MFP can handle tracking your daily weight measurements.

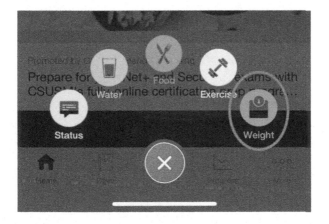

MFP also gives you the option to take photos, which I highly recommend, when you go to record your weight.

Pictures, along with mirror reflection analysis, will help you get a better understanding of how you're progressing. It's also really great to look back at your old photos and compare them with the new you! MFP lets you compare photos side by side, detailing both the date you took the picture and how much you weighed in that day.

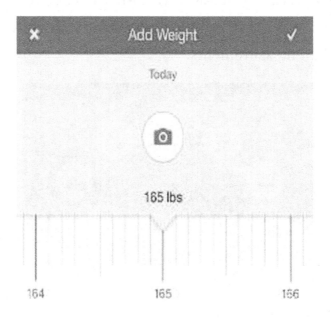

If you'd like to see your progress, at a glance, you can do so by selecting *Progress* in MFP's lower menu.

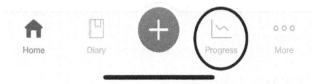

Selecting this will take you to a page where you can view the progress you've made. It allows you to view your past progress in a graph mode. The graph shows data points for your weight entries (the y-axis) and the date you recorded them (x-axis). You can also adjust the time frame of this graph by weeks, months, and years.

This is a handy feature that is much better than keeping a separate journal and having to write down measurements every day in my opinion. Either way, be consistent, and your graph will end up looking like a beautiful fluctuating mess.

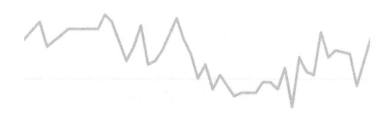

After recording your weight for the day, continue with step #2.

## 2. Measure your waist

Now, I want you to measure your waist (around the navel) once a week on the same day after you've weighed yourself.

A tape measure is arguably more revealing than the scale because you can potentially have a smaller waist on the same day the weight on the scale is stagnant.

Along with photos, it can be a determining factor, to check, if you've truly gained weight or if your body is just retaining water. For those reasons, it's a good idea to measure your waist, just above the belly button, after you weigh in.

To get the most accurate reading, relax and don't suck in your tummy. Breathe as you normally would and get a reading.

MFP will track waist measurements in the same fashion it tracks weight.

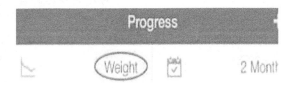

You can change the progress settings by switching "Weight" to "Waist" to record your waist measurement.

You can choose to write this down in your training log as well. Now that you've written everything down (weight and waist), **what you're going to do is take weekly averages.**

Remember, only take your weight averages. Measure your waist once a week on the same day.

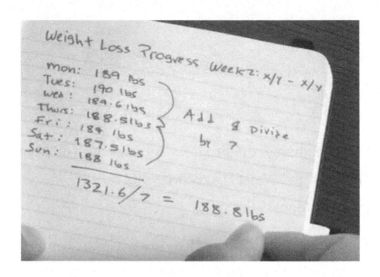

*Above is an example of how you would track your weight loss progress. At the end of the week, you add up all your weigh-ins and divide by 7 —*
*that's how you get your weekly average **(I've included a spreadsheet in the bonus course that does this for you).***

Here are a couple of scenarios that you should know when assessing the numbers.

**Scenario 1:**

If your weekly averages are going down, then you're in good shape. Keep doing what you're doing.

**Scenario 2:**

If your weekly weight average is not going down, but your waist measurement is going down, then you're in good shape also. This can mean you're losing fat and building muscle at the same time! Beginners will experience this most often.

**Scenario 3:**

If both of your weekly averages are NOT going down and even going up, then you're doing something wrong. It can be for any of the reasons described before, or it could be that you're not tracking correctly.

You can try decreasing calories from carbohydrates or move more as described above under "Activity." If you fall into the category of scenario 3, then you have to adjust something. Weight loss, as we know, is all about calories in vs.

calories out. There are no exceptions to this rule. **If you're stalling, then you're NOT burning more calories than you consume.**

You MAY need a refeed day or cheat meal in this case to help boost leptin. Refer to the FAQ meal planning section for more information on this.

For most people, plateauing can be very frustrating — especially if you were extremely close to reaching your weight loss goals. However, plateauing does not always have to be a bad thing. If anything, it should be taken as a sign of great progress!

Plateauing means that your body fat has reduced notably and that you are well on your way to a leaner physique. Therefore, the key in this instance is to keep eating at a deficit and if possible, increase your physical activity levels. (Note: your deficit may also require tweaking.) In no time, you will see the fruits of your labor as the numbers on the scale start dropping again!

# Final Thoughts on IIFYM!

IIFYM is an amazingly effective dieting technique; I hope I've convinced you of that. For us fitness folks, we know that getting to our dream physique takes a lot of hard work. IIFYM is one way to help us reach our goal.

I'm sure by now you know that the human body is a finely tuned piece of biological machinery. It'll let go of fat when enough energy is demanded (a caloric deficit + exercise demands that your body digs into your fat stores for energy). **If you keep pushing it, your body composition will have no choice but to change when you follow the IIFYM principles taught in this book.**

IIFYM will separate you from the pack. It'll keep you from "guessing your way to weight loss" like the rest of the world does. By taking the time to apply IIFYM to you weight loss goals, you'll get real, long lasting, results. I hope this book plays a role in getting you to the body and health you've always wanted.

# Bonus Chapter

I've decided to include this bonus chapter which goes over a few tips on what to do when you have a social event coming up or when you're stuck eating at a fast-food joint, or any similar scenario (I know, it happens). Let me show you how to mitigate the damage.

### Fast-Food, Fat-Loss Guide

I remember when I used to be so strict with my dieting. I would say "No, I can't tonight. No macros/calories left," whenever someone asked me to go out to eat or if I was invited out to a night on the town. **I would even say no to my mom's birthday cake!**

How sad is that? What's the point of losing weight if you can't even eat out at restaurants and enjoy your favorite foods, let alone, your mom's birthday cake!? Dieting shouldn't just be about eating chicken, broccoli, and brown rice. It should be about knowing how to wisely choose and plan out your meals so that you can eat enjoyably and more importantly, guilt-free.

## How to Eat "Dirty" Foods, Guilt-Free

Make sure to check out your free course, found at the end of the book, to see how to add fast-food to MFP and track your macros.

## Scenario 1: If you know you have an event/date/night out/etc. coming up.

Let's say you have a wedding coming up (not yours). You know there's going to be a sh** ton of food and delicious cake. What do you do? It's simple: you can utilize intermittent fasting for that day.

Intermittent fasting in a nutshell:

- Push your first meal back 4-6 hours after waking.
- Utilize black coffee and/or sparkling water to make the fast easy to get through.

Now, here's what to do:

1. You can either fast until the wedding begins and eat all your calories at the wedding. This wouldn't be my choice, but it does work, so long as you don't overdo it.

2. You could fast as you normally would, however, you would eat 1-2 meals prior that consist only of protein and veggies. *This would be my choice.* With this option, you would hit all your protein macros easier, which matters when trying to lose weight, and it doesn't take up many calories.

You'll still feel somewhat satiated due to the protein and you'll still have room for the "feast" at the wedding. This works also for a date, where you know you're going to eat out at a restaurant. Simply extend your fast or keep your biggest meal for last. If you're going out to the club or just happen to find yourself going to a fast-food joint at 3 in the morning **(trust me, I've been there)**, there are a couple of macro-friendly options you can choose as well.

**Here are a few places that I've found to have great macros:**

*Note: Not all of these macros are 100% accurate due to the different serving sizes the person gives you. Also, there's will always be an updated list in the course, whenever I find more options.*

### #1 Panda Express

*Panda Express's Chicken Teriyaki has a crazy amount of protein.*

What I usually get is the following:

**Option 1:** Double Chicken Teriyaki, Half Steamed Veggies, Half White Rice.
**Macros:** *825 Cal, 78g protein, 66g carbs, 26g fat*

*Option 2:* Double Chicken Teriyaki, Half Steamed Veggies, Half Brown Rice.
*Macros:* *860 Cal, 79g protein, 69g carbs, 29g fat*

***Option 3:*** *Double Chicken Teriyaki, Full Steamed Veggies*
***Macros:*** *680 Cal, 76g protein, 32g carbs, 27g fat*

## #2 El Pollo Loco

El Pollo Loco is another place that offers crazy amounts of protein with most of their 2 & 3-piece combos.

## Personal favorite out of everything on this list: 3-piece combo - 2 Skinless Chicken Breast, 1 Wing. Sides: Broccoli & Pinto Beans
***Macros:*** *675 Cal, 96g protein, 35g carbs, 16g fat*

## #3 Chipotle

There are endless amounts of options for chipotle so I will not list them all here but, these are my personal favorites.

**Option 1:** Burrito Bowl (Double Meat):  Chicken, Barbacoa, White Rice, Fajita Vegetables, Mild Salsa, Cheese, Lettuce

**Marcos:** *1015 Cal, 71g protein, 99g carbs, 38g fat*

**Option 2:** Burrito (Double Meat - usually only eat this if I'm bulking or if I have a lot of calories left):

Chicken, Steak, Brown Rice, White Rice, Black Beans, Fajita Vegetables, Fresh Tomato Salsa, Corn Salsa, Sour Cream, Cheese, Guac, Lettuce

**Macros:** *1550 Cal, 88g protein, 146g carbs, 70g fat*

**Option 3:** Burrito Bowl (Usually only eat this if I'm cutting or if I don't have many calories left): Double Chicken, Fajita Vegetables, Corn Salsa, Cheese, Guac, Lettuce

**Macros:** *795 Cal, 74g protein, 30g carb, 46g fat*

## #4 Chick-fil-a

**Option 1:** Two Grilled Chicken Sandwiches
**Macros:** *640 Cal, 60g protein, 80g carbs, 10g fat*

**Option 2:** 12 Piece Grilled Nuggets (Not Including sauces)
 **Macros:** *210 Cal, 38g protein, 3g carbs, 5g fat*

## #5 McDonald's

**Option 1**: 10 Piece Chicken Nuggets
*Macros:* 440 Cal, 24g protein, 26g carbs, 27g fat

**Option 2:** 4 Piece Buttermilk Crispy Tenders
**Macros:** *500 Cal, 39g protein, 25g carbs, 27g fat*

**Option 3:** Bacon Ranch Grilled Chicken Salad
**Macros:** *320 Cal, 42g protein, 9g carbs, 14g fat*

## #6 Tacobell

**Option 1:** Crunchy Taco with Shredded Chicken
**Macros:** *160 Cal, 9g protein, 11g carbs, 8g fat*

**Option 2:** Power Menu Burrito – Chicken
**Macros:** *450 Cal, 26g protein, 41g carbs, 20g fat*

**Option 3:** Power Menu Bowl – Chicken
**Macros:** *500 Cal, 27g protein, 54g carbs, 20g fat*

## #7 Starbucks

**Option 1:** Caffe Americano
**Macros:** *0 Cal*

**Option 2:** Skinny Vanilla Latte
**Macros:** *130 Cal, 12g protein, 19g carbs, 0g fat*

**Option 3:** Teavana® Shaken Iced Passion Tango™ Tea
**Macros:** *45 Cal, 0g protein, 11g carbs, 0g fat*

**Option 4:** Non-Fat Green Tea Latte
**Macros:** *240 Cal, 12g protein, 34g carbs, 7g fat*

**Scenario 2: When an unplanned event occurs, and you didn't save up any calories/macros/etc.**

This scenario has a simple fix as well. Just accept it. Shit happens. Life happens.

Unless you're competing for a competition, there is no need to worry about a one-night binge.

Like Brandon Carter says, and I'm paraphrasing here:

*"One night of bad eating is not going to make you fat, just like one night of 'good' eating is going to make you ripped."*

Are you really going to say no to your mom's cooking every-time? Let's be realistic here.

Now, if you go WAY overboard and eat like 3000-5000+ extra calories than you're supposed to, then maybe you should probably do a few extra cardio sessions that week and eat slightly less for a day or two.

But if you went over 200-600 calories over... who cares? Just get back to it the next day and don't beat yourself up over it. It's about sticking to the process. If you're sticking to it 95% of the time, you'll be fine.

If implemented correctly, flexible dieting can easily become the gift that keeps on giving. It is easy to adapt to, and not for short-term weight loss goals, but also for long-term lifestyle changes that maintain a healthier lifestyle and a fitter body!

# One Last Thing...

*"No, the journey doesn't end here. Death is just another path. One that we all must take."* - *Gandalf*

*Wow, that's a deep quote for a last reminder. Sorry about that. My inner geek had to come out sooner or later!*

Anyways, if I've been successful with this book, the IIFYM strategy should be crystal clear. You should know more about the basics of nutrition than 95% of others around you and you should be on your way to achieving your best body ever. Yet, we all know that you have to take action to see results. **Don't put this off another week or until tomorrow.** Start now and track the macros of your next meal. Even if it's something as small as inputting a banana into MyFitnessPal. Do it now. It's a small step towards massive success. Soon, tracking macros will be second nature and you'll never look back.

# Thank You!

Dear friend,

It's Christian here. Before you go, I'd just like to say thank you purchasing my book. I know that if you follow what you've learned, you'll see a ton of success in your fitness journey.

Would you do me a favor and pass the word along to your friends to help them focus on their fat loss goals, too? IIFYM is much more than a way to lose weight. It's a lifestyle.

Also, if you've received any value from this book, would you mind taking a minute to give me feedback in the form of a review on Amazon about this book? I'm an independent writer and self-published this book on Amazon. I love to keep improving and you leaving a review can help me make this book even better. You can leave me a review by visiting:

### *Bit.ly/iifym-book-review*

I'd also like to share some bonus resources with you to help you in your fitness journey. Get them at *iifymbook.club*

And one last thing, send me an email (christian@leanwithstyle.com, subject: my IIFYM life), and let me know one thing you learned or loved about this book. I'd love to hear from you.

To your success,
Christian Pinedo

**P.S.**

*If you ever want to reach out with a question, or see what I'm doing, reach out to me on Instagram via Direct Message (DM):*

### *@chris_pinedo*

*You can also find me on my YouTube Channel:*

### *@Chris Pinedo*

*I regularly upload videos all about IIFYM, Fat Loss, Strength Training, and a whole lot more. I'd love to see you there!*

# References

1.  "Low calorie dieting increases cortisol. - NCBI - NIH." 5 Apr. 2010, https://www.ncbi.nlm.nih.gov/pubmed/20368473.

2.  "Rigid vs. flexible dieting: association with eating disorder symptoms in ...." https://www.ncbi.nlm.nih.gov/pubmed/11883916.

3.  https://bodyrecomposition.com/fat-loss/how-to-estimate-maintenance-caloric-intake.html/

4.  "Inadequate dietary protein increases hunger and desire to eat in ...." https://www.ncbi.nlm.nih.gov/pubmed/17513410.

5.  "Diet induced thermogenesis measured over 24h in a ... - Nature." https://www.nature.com/ijo/journal/v23/n3/pdf/0800810a.pdf?origin=ppub.

6.  "Glycogen storage capacity and de novo lipogenesis during massive ...." https://www.ncbi.nlm.nih.gov/pubmed/3165600.

7.  "Effect of two different weight-loss rates on body composition ... - NCBI." https://www.ncbi.nlm.nih.gov/pubmed/21558571.

8. "Macronutrient content of a hypoenergy diet affects nitrogen retention ...."
https://www.ncbi.nlm.nih.gov/pubmed/3182156.

9. https://www.fda.gov/Food/GuidanceRegulation/GuidanceDocumentsRegulatoryInformation/LabelingNutrition/ucm053479.htm

10. "Exercise and the Institute of Medicine recommendations for nutrition.."
https://www.ncbi.nlm.nih.gov/pubmed/16004827.

11. "The myths surrounding pre-exercise carbohydrate feeding. - NCBI." 22 Feb. 2011,
https://www.ncbi.nlm.nih.gov/pubmed/21346333.

12. "Ingested protein dose response of muscle and albumin protein ... - NCBI." 3 Dec. 2008,
https://www.ncbi.nlm.nih.gov/pubmed/19056590.

13. "Leptin signaling, adiposity, and energy balance. - NCBI."
https://www.ncbi.nlm.nih.gov/pubmed/12079865.

Made in the USA
Monee, IL
03 January 2021